MENSTRUAL CRAMPS RELIEF COOKBOOK

Dr. Kimberly Carlos

Copyright © 2023 by Dr. Kimberly Carlos

TABLE OF CONTENT

INTRODUCTION

Sarah had always struggled with excruciating menstrual cramps that left her bedridden every month. She had tried countless painkillers and remedies, but nothing seemed to offer lasting relief.

Frustration and discomfort were her constant companions during that time of the month.

One day, while scrolling through her social media feed, Sarah stumbled upon a post about a menstrual cramps relief diet. Skeptical yet desperate for relief, she decided to give it a try. She researched the recommended foods, making a shopping list filled with nutrient-rich options like leafy greens, fatty fish, and fruits.

For the first month, Sarah diligently followed the diet, replacing her usual junk food cravings with wholesome alternatives. She incorporated ginger tea into her daily routine and swapped sugary snacks for nuts and seeds. Slowly but surely, she started noticing a difference.

The next menstrual cycle arrived, and Sarah braced herself for the usual agony.

To her surprise, the cramps were milder, and her mood swings were less severe. The diet seemed to be working. Encouraged by the improvement, Sarah continued with her new eating habits and even included regular exercise in her routine.

Over time, the relief was remarkable. The menstrual cramps that once immobilized her had become manageable, allowing her to live a more active and enjoyable life. Sarah shared her success with her friends and online communities, hoping to help others find comfort during their periods.

Sarah's story became an inspiration for many, proving that sometimes, relief can be found in the most unexpected places – like a simple, mindful, and nutritious diet tailored to one's unique needs.

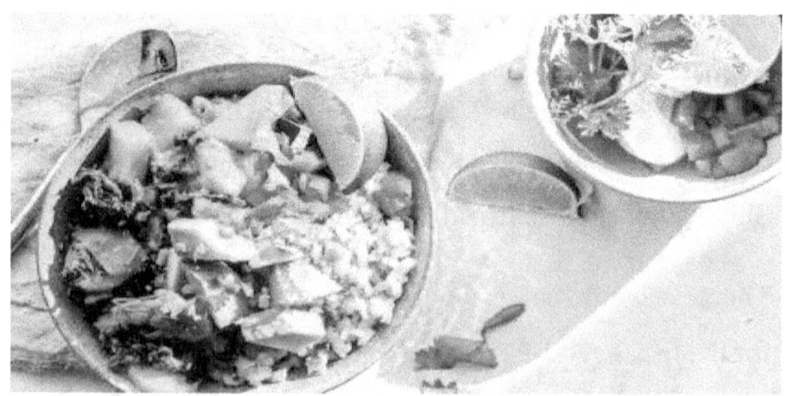

CHAPTER ONE

Following a Menstrual Cramps Relief Diet with Benefits

Following a menstrual cramps relief diet can help alleviate discomfort and improve your overall well-being during your period. Here are some steps to follow such a diet with benefits:

1. Research and Plan:

- Start by researching foods that are known to help relieve menstrual cramps. Focus on nutrient-rich, anti-inflammatory options.
- Create a meal plan that includes these foods. Consider consulting a registered dietitian for personalized guidance.

2. Incorporate Nutrient-Rich Foods:

- Include foods high in vitamins and minerals like magnesium, calcium, and vitamin D, which can help reduce cramps. Examples include leafy greens, dairy or dairy alternatives, and fatty fish.
- Consume iron-rich foods to combat fatigue and

replenish blood lost during your period, such as lean meats, beans, and fortified cereals.

3. Anti-Inflammatory Foods:

- Opt for anti-inflammatory foods to reduce inflammation and pain. This includes fruits (especially berries), vegetables, whole grains, and healthy fats like olive oil and avocados.
- Ginger and turmeric are known for their anti-inflammatory properties; consider incorporating them into your diet through teas, smoothies, or cooking.

4. Stay Hydrated: Drink plenty of water to stay hydrated, which can help alleviate bloating and cramps.

5. Fiber-Rich Foods: High-fiber foods like whole grains, beans, and vegetables can help regulate bowel movements and reduce constipation, which is often exacerbated during menstruation.

6. Limit Caffeine and Sugary Foods: Caffeine and sugary foods can exacerbate cramps and mood swings. Try to reduce your intake of coffee, soda, and sweets.

7. Mindful Eating: Pay attention to your body's signals. Eat slowly and mindfully, and stop when you're full.

8. Herbal Teas: Herbal teas like chamomile, peppermint, and raspberry leaf may offer relief from cramps. Experiment with different types and see which works best for you.

9. Regular Exercise: Engage in regular physical activity throughout your menstrual cycle. Exercise can help alleviate cramps by increasing blood flow and releasing endorphins.

10. Supplements: Consult with a healthcare professional about the potential benefits of supplements like magnesium, calcium, or omega-3 fatty acids in your specific case.

11. Maintain a Balanced Diet Beyond Your Period: Don't just focus on these foods during your period; incorporate them into your regular diet for long-term benefits.

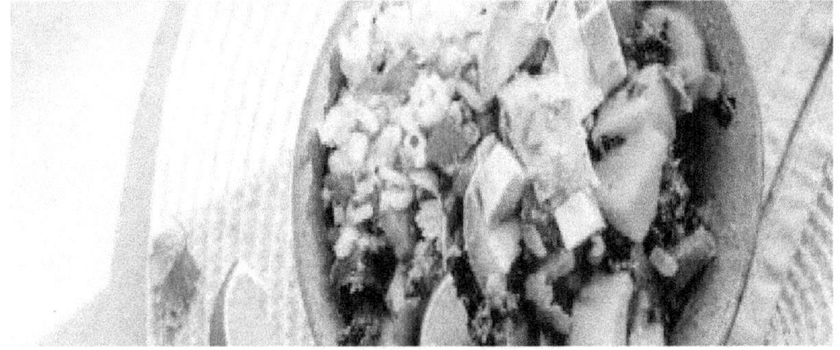

12. Track Your Progress: Keep a journal to track your menstrual cycles, symptoms, and dietary changes. This can help you identify which foods and habits work best for you.

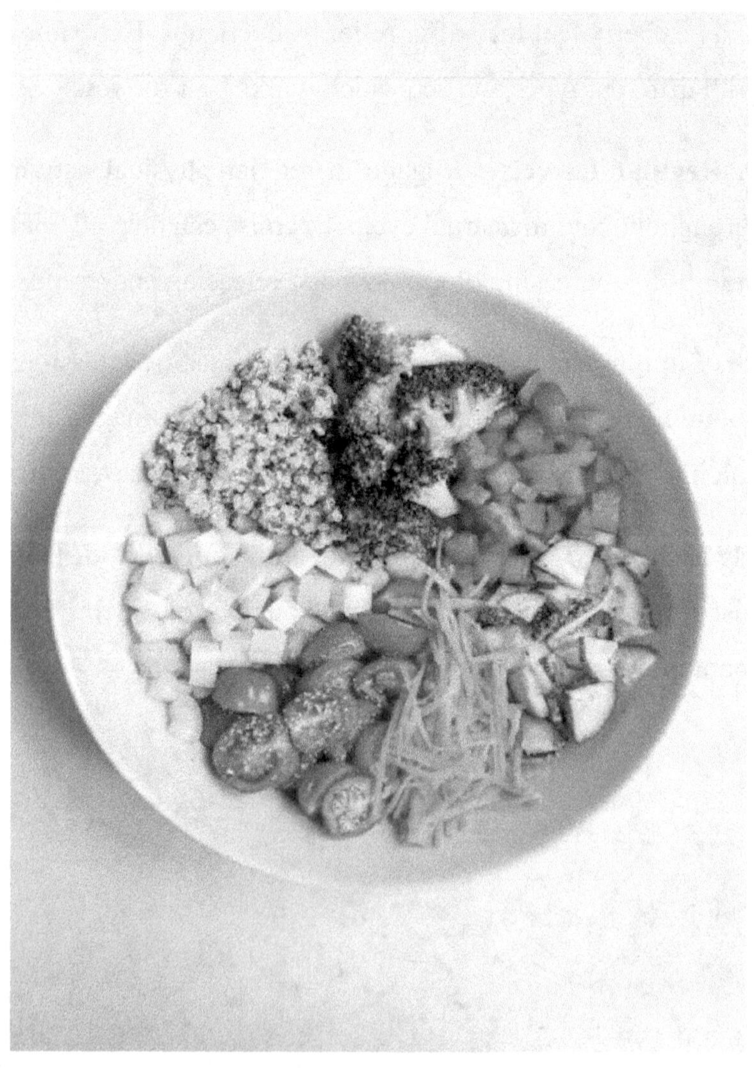

CHAPTER TWO

14-Day Menstrual Cramps Relief Diet Meal Plan

Day 1:

- Breakfast: Greek yogurt with mixed berries and a sprinkle of chia seeds.
- Lunch: Spinach and kale salad with grilled chicken, avocado, and olive oil vinaigrette.
- Snack: Carrot and cucumber sticks with hummus.
- Dinner: Baked salmon with quinoa and steamed broccoli.

Day 2:

- Breakfast: Oatmeal topped with sliced banana, almonds, and a drizzle of honey.
- Lunch: Lentil soup with a side of whole-grain bread and a green salad.
- Snack: Greek yogurt with honey and a handful of walnuts.
- Dinner: Stir-fried tofu with mixed vegetables and brown rice.

Day 3:

- Breakfast: Smoothie with spinach, pineapple, ginger, and chia seeds.
- Lunch: Quinoa and black bean salad with roasted sweet potatoes and a lime-cilantro dressing.
- Snack: Sliced apple with almond butter.
- Dinner: Grilled shrimp with quinoa and steamed asparagus.

Day 4:

- Breakfast: Scrambled eggs with spinach and feta cheese.
- Lunch: Chickpea and vegetable curry with brown rice.
- Snack: Mixed nuts and dried fruits.
- Dinner: Baked chicken breast with roasted Brussels sprouts and quinoa.

Day 5:

- Breakfast: Whole-grain toast with mashed avocado and poached eggs.
- Lunch: Spinach and arugula salad with grilled salmon, cherry tomatoes, and balsamic vinaigrette.

- Snack: Sliced cucumber with tzatziki sauce.

- Dinner: Quinoa-stuffed bell peppers with a side of steamed broccoli.

Day 6:

- Breakfast: Overnight oats with almond milk, strawberries, and a sprinkle of flaxseed.

- Lunch: Lentil and vegetable stir-fry with brown rice.

- Snack: Sliced pear with a handful of cashews.

- Dinner: Baked cod with quinoa and sautéed spinach.

Day 7:

- Breakfast: Whole-grain pancakes with Greek yogurt and mixed berries.

- Lunch: Spinach and feta stuffed chicken breast with roasted sweet potatoes.

- Snack: Baby carrots with tzatziki dip.

- Dinner: Beef and vegetable kebabs with quinoa and a side of green beans.

Day 8:

- Breakfast: Scrambled tofu with sautéed spinach, bell peppers, and a sprinkle of nutritional yeast.

- Lunch: Quinoa and black bean salad with diced avocado and a squeeze of lime.
- Snack: Sliced apple with a dollop of almond butter.
- Dinner: Grilled shrimp with quinoa and steamed asparagus.

Day 9:

- Breakfast: Smoothie with kale, banana, almond milk, and a scoop of plant-based protein powder.
- Lunch: Chickpea and vegetable curry with brown rice.
- Snack: Mixed nuts and dried fruits.
- Dinner: Baked chicken breast with roasted Brussels sprouts and quinoa.

Day 10:

- Breakfast: Whole-grain toast with mashed avocado and poached eggs.
- Lunch: Spinach and arugula salad with grilled salmon, cherry tomatoes, and balsamic vinaigrette.
- Snack: Sliced cucumber with tzatziki sauce.
- Dinner: Quinoa-stuffed bell peppers with a side of steamed broccoli.

Day 11:

- Breakfast: Overnight oats with almond milk, strawberries, and a sprinkle of flaxseed.
- Lunch: Lentil and vegetable stir-fry with brown rice.
- Snack: Sliced pear with a handful of cashews.
- Dinner: Baked cod with quinoa and sautéed spinach.

Day 12:

- Breakfast: Whole-grain pancakes with Greek yogurt and mixed berries.
- Lunch: Spinach and feta stuffed chicken breast with roasted sweet potatoes.
- Snack: Baby carrots with tzatziki dip.
- Dinner: Beef and vegetable kebabs with quinoa and a side of green beans.

Day 13:

- Breakfast: Greek yogurt with mixed berries and a sprinkle of chia seeds.
- Lunch: Spinach and kale salad with grilled chicken, avocado, and olive oil vinaigrette.
- Snack: Carrot and cucumber sticks with hummus.
- Dinner: Baked salmon with quinoa and steamed

broccoli.

Day 14:

- Breakfast: Oatmeal topped with sliced banana, almonds, and a drizzle of honey.
- Lunch: Lentil soup with a side of whole-grain bread and a green salad.
- Snack: Greek yogurt with honey and a handful of walnuts.
- Dinner: Stir-fried tofu with mixed vegetables and brown rice.

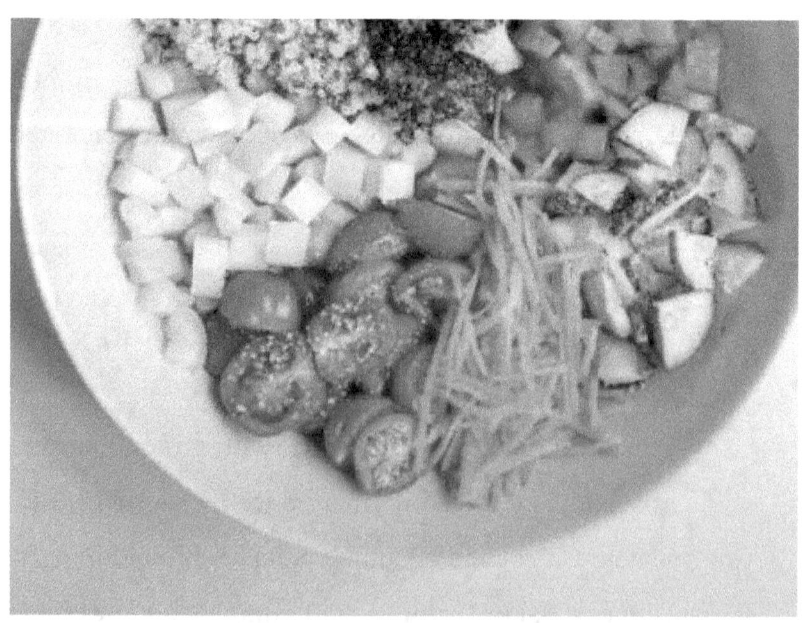

CHAPTER THREE

Menstrual Cramp Relief Diet Breakfast Recipes

1. Berry and Spinach Smoothie

This smoothie is packed with nutrients like iron and antioxidants from spinach and berries, which can help alleviate cramps.

Ingredients:

- 1 cup fresh spinach leaves
- 1/2 cup mixed berries (e.g., strawberries, blueberries, raspberries)
- 1 banana
- 1/2 cup Greek yogurt
- 1 tablespoon honey (optional)
- 1/2 cup almond milk

Instructions:

1. Add all the ingredients to a blender.

2. Blend until smooth.

3. Pour into a glass and enjoy!

Cooking Time: 5 minutes

2. Almond Butter and Banana Toast

This quick and nutritious breakfast provides magnesium and potassium from bananas and healthy fats from almond butter, which can help reduce cramping.

Ingredients:

- 2 slices whole-grain bread
- 2 tablespoons almond butter
- 1 ripe banana, sliced

Instructions:

1. Toast the bread to your preferred level of crispiness.

2. Spread almond butter evenly on each slice.

3. Arrange banana slices on top.

4. Serve and enjoy!

Cooking Time: 5 minutes

3. Greek Yogurt Parfait

This parfait is rich in calcium from Greek yogurt, which may help ease cramps, and is topped with fruits and nuts for added nutrition.

Ingredients:

- 1 cup Greek yogurt
- 1/2 cup mixed berries
- 2 tablespoons granola
- 1 tablespoon honey (optional)

Instructions:

1. In a glass or bowl, layer Greek yogurt, mixed berries, and granola.

2. Drizzle with honey if desired.

3. Repeat for additional servings.

4. Dig in!

Cooking Time: 5 minutes

4. Scrambled Tofu with Spinach

Tofu provides plant-based protein, while spinach offers iron, making this breakfast perfect for cramp relief.

Ingredients:

- 1/2 block firm tofu, crumbled

- 1 cup fresh spinach leaves
- 1/2 teaspoon turmeric
- Salt and pepper to taste
- 1 teaspoon olive oil

Instructions:

1. Heat olive oil in a pan over medium heat.

2. Add crumbled tofu and turmeric; sauté for 2-3 minutes.

3. Stir in spinach and cook until wilted.

4. Season with salt and pepper.

5. Serve hot!

Cooking Time: 10 minutes

5. Banana and Spinach Pancakes

These pancakes incorporate spinach for added nutrients and are topped with banana slices for a cramp-relieving boost.

Ingredients:

- 1 cup spinach leaves
- 1 ripe banana

- 1 cup pancake mix

- 1/2 cup almond milk

Instructions:

1. In a blender, combine spinach, banana, and almond milk; blend until smooth.

2. Mix the green smoothie with pancake mix until well combined.

3. Cook pancakes on a griddle or non-stick pan until golden brown.

4. Serve with extra banana slices.

Cooking Time: 15 minutes

6. Chia Seed Pudding with Berries

Chia seeds are packed with fiber and omega-3s, which can help reduce inflammation and cramps.

Ingredients:

- 2 tablespoons chia seeds

- 1/2 cup almond milk

- 1/2 cup mixed berries

- 1 teaspoon honey (optional)

Instructions:

1. In a jar or bowl, mix chia seeds and almond milk.

2. Stir well, then refrigerate for at least 2 hours or overnight to thicken.

3. Top with mixed berries and honey.

4. Enjoy your chia pudding!

Cooking Time: 2 hours (mostly refrigeration time)

7. Avocado and Tomato Toast

This toast features avocado for healthy fats and tomatoes for vitamin C, which can help ease cramps.

Ingredients:

- 2 slices whole-grain bread
- 1 ripe avocado, mashed
- 1 small tomato, sliced
- Salt and pepper to taste

Instructions:

1. Toast the bread to your preference.

2. Spread mashed avocado evenly on each slice.

3. Top with sliced tomatoes.

4. Season with salt and pepper.

5. Serve and enjoy!

Cooking Time: 5 minutes

8. Quinoa Breakfast Bowl

Quinoa is high in magnesium and protein, which can help reduce muscle tension and cramps.

Ingredients:

- 1/2 cup cooked quinoa
- 1/4 cup Greek yogurt
- 1/4 cup mixed berries
- 1 tablespoon honey
- 1 tablespoon chopped nuts (e.g., almonds or walnuts)

Instructions:

1. In a bowl, layer quinoa, Greek yogurt, mixed berries, and nuts.

2. Drizzle with honey.

3. Mix well and savor your quinoa bowl!

Cooking Time: 10 minutes (if quinoa is pre-cooked)

9. Sweet Potato and Spinach Breakfast Hash

Sweet potatoes provide complex carbohydrates and vitamin A, while spinach offers iron, making this a nourishing cramp-relief breakfast.

Ingredients:

- 1 small sweet potato, diced
- 1 cup fresh spinach leaves
- 1/2 small red onion, diced
- 1/2 teaspoon paprika
- Salt and pepper to taste
- 1 teaspoon olive oil

Instructions:

1. Heat olive oil in a pan over medium heat.

2. Add sweet potato and onion; sauté for 7-8 minutes until tender.

3. Stir in spinach and cook until wilted.

4. Season with paprika, salt, and pepper.

5. Serve hot!

Cooking Time: 15 minutes

10. Peanut Butter and Banana Smoothie Bowl

This smoothie bowl is a creamy and satisfying breakfast that combines potassium from bananas and protein from peanut butter.

Ingredients:

- 2 ripe bananas, frozen
- 2 tablespoons peanut butter
- 1/2 cup almond milk
- Toppings: sliced banana, chia seeds, and a drizzle of honey (optional)

Instructions:

1. Blend frozen bananas, peanut butter, and almond milk until smooth.

2. Pour into a bowl.

3. Top with banana slices, chia seeds, and honey if desired.

4. Enjoy your smoothie bowl with a spoon!

Cooking Time: 5 minutes

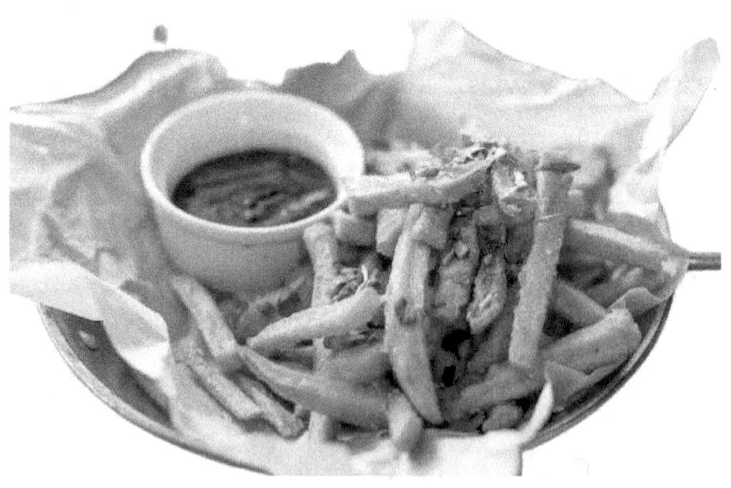

Menstrual Cramp Relief Diet Lunch Recipes

1. Spinach and Chickpea Salad

This salad is rich in iron from spinach and protein from chickpeas, which can help reduce cramps.

Ingredients:

- 2 cups fresh spinach leaves
- 1 cup canned chickpeas, drained and rinsed
- 1/2 cucumber, sliced
- 1/4 red onion, thinly sliced
- 1/4 cup feta cheese (optional)
- Balsamic vinaigrette dressing

Instructions:

1. In a salad bowl, combine spinach, chickpeas, cucumber, and red onion.

2. Top with feta cheese if desired.

3. Drizzle with balsamic vinaigrette dressing.

4. Toss gently and enjoy!

Cooking Time: 10 minutes (no cooking required)

2. Quinoa and Black Bean Bowl

This bowl combines quinoa for magnesium and black beans for protein, both of which can help relieve cramps.

Ingredients:

- 1 cup cooked quinoa
- 1/2 cup canned black beans, drained and rinsed
- 1/2 red bell pepper, diced
- 1/2 avocado, sliced
- Lime-cilantro dressing

Instructions:

1. In a bowl, layer cooked quinoa, black beans, red bell pepper, and avocado slices.

2. Drizzle with lime-cilantro dressing.

3. Mix well and savor!

Cooking Time: 10 minutes (if quinoa is pre-cooked)

3. Salmon and Asparagus

This simple yet nutritious lunch features salmon for omega-3 fatty acids and asparagus for its anti-inflammatory properties.

Ingredients:

- 2 salmon fillets
- 1 bunch asparagus, trimmed
- 1 lemon, sliced
- Olive oil
- Salt and pepper to taste

Instructions:

1. Preheat your oven to 375°F (190°C).

2. Place salmon fillets and asparagus on a baking sheet.

3. Drizzle with olive oil, season with salt and pepper, and add lemon slices.

4. Bake for 15-20 minutes or until salmon is cooked through.

5. Serve hot!

 Cooking Time: 20-25 minutes

4. Lentil and Vegetable Soup

This hearty soup is loaded with lentils for iron and various vegetables for nutrients, making it a great choice for cramp relief.

Ingredients:

- 1 cup dried green or brown lentils
- 4 cups vegetable broth
- 1 onion, chopped
- 2 carrots, sliced
- 2 celery stalks, sliced
- 1 cup diced tomatoes
- 1 teaspoon dried thyme
- Salt and pepper to taste

Instructions:

1. In a large pot, sauté the onion, carrots, and celery until softened.

2. Add lentils, vegetable broth, diced tomatoes, thyme, salt, and pepper.

3. Simmer for about 30 minutes or until lentils are tender.

4. Serve your comforting lentil soup!

Cooking Time: 40-45 minutes

5. Tofu and Vegetable Stir-Fry

This stir-fry features tofu for protein and an array of colorful vegetables, providing essential nutrients to ease menstrual cramps.

Ingredients:

- 1/2 block firm tofu, cubed
- 2 cups mixed vegetables (e.g., bell peppers, broccoli, carrots)
- 2 tablespoons soy sauce
- 1 tablespoon sesame oil
- 1 teaspoon ginger, minced
- Cooked brown rice

Instructions:

1. Heat sesame oil in a pan or wok over medium-high heat.

2. Add tofu and stir-fry until golden.

3. Add mixed vegetables and ginger; stir-fry until tender-crisp.

4. Stir in soy sauce.

5. Serve over cooked brown rice.

Cooking Time: 15 minutes

6. Spinach and Feta Stuffed Chicken Breast

This dish pairs lean protein from chicken with iron-rich spinach, and feta for flavor, offering cramp relief in a delicious package.

Ingredients:

- 2 boneless, skinless chicken breasts
- 2 cups fresh spinach leaves
- 1/4 cup crumbled feta cheese
- Salt and pepper to taste
- Olive oil

Instructions:

1. Preheat your oven to 375°F (190°C).

2. Slice a pocket into each chicken breast.

3. Stuff each breast with spinach and feta cheese.

4. Season with salt and pepper.

5. Heat olive oil in an ovenproof skillet, then sear chicken for 2-3 minutes per side.

6. Transfer the skillet to the oven and bake for 20-25 minutes or until chicken is cooked through.

7. Serve hot!

Cooking Time: 30-35 minutes

7. Chickpea and Avocado Wrap

This wrap combines chickpeas for fiber and avocado for healthy fats, offering a satisfying and cramp-relieving lunch option.

Ingredients:

- 1 whole-grain tortilla or wrap
- 1/2 cup canned chickpeas, mashed
- 1/2 avocado, sliced
- Baby spinach leaves
- Sliced red bell pepper
- Hummus (optional)

Instructions:

1. Lay the tortilla flat.

2. Spread mashed chickpeas on the tortilla.

3. Top with avocado slices, spinach leaves, and red bell pepper strips.

4. Optionally, add a drizzle of hummus.

5. Roll up the wrap and enjoy!

Cooking Time: 5 minutes (no cooking required)

8. Shrimp and Quinoa Salad

This salad combines shrimp for protein and quinoa for magnesium, making it a nourishing option for cramp relief.

Ingredients:

- 1 cup cooked quinoa
- 1/2 pound cooked shrimp, peeled and deveined
- 1 cup cherry tomatoes, halved
- 1/2 cucumber, diced
- Fresh basil leaves
- Lemon-tahini dressing

Instructions:

1. In a salad bowl, combine quinoa, cooked shrimp, cherry tomatoes, cucumber, and fresh basil leaves.

2. Drizzle with lemon-tahini dressing.

3. Toss gently and enjoy!

Cooking Time: 15 minutes (if quinoa and shrimp are pre-cooked)

9. Sweet Potato and Black Bean Bowl

This bowl features sweet potatoes for complex carbohydrates and black beans for protein, offering cramp relief and a satisfying lunch.

Ingredients:

- 1 medium sweet potato, diced
- 1 cup cooked black beans
- 1/2 cup corn kernels (fresh, frozen, or canned)
- 1/4 cup diced red onion
- 1/4 cup chopped cilantro
- Lime wedges

Instructions:

1. Roast sweet potato cubes in the oven at 375°F (190°C) for about 20 minutes or until tender.

2. In a bowl, combine roasted sweet potatoes, black beans, corn, red onion, and cilantro.

3. Serve with lime wedges for added zing.

Cooking Time: 20-25 minutes

10. Mediterranean Quinoa Salad

This Mediterranean-inspired salad combines quinoa for magnesium and a variety of colorful vegetables and olives for added nutrients.

Ingredients:

- 1 cup cooked quinoa
- Cherry tomatoes, halved
- Cucumber slices
- Kalamata olives, pitted
- Red onion, thinly sliced
- Feta cheese (optional)
- Greek salad dressing

Instructions:

1. In a salad bowl, combine cooked quinoa, cherry tomatoes, cucumber slices, Kalamata olives, and red onion.

2. Add crumbled feta cheese if desired.

3. Drizzle with Greek salad dressing.

4. Toss gently and enjoy your Mediterranean quinoa salad!

Cooking Time: 15 minutes (if quinoa is pre-cooked)

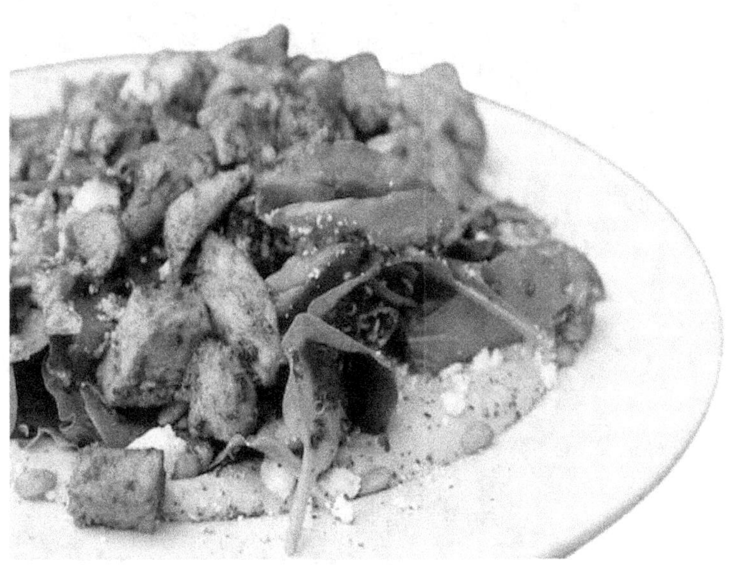

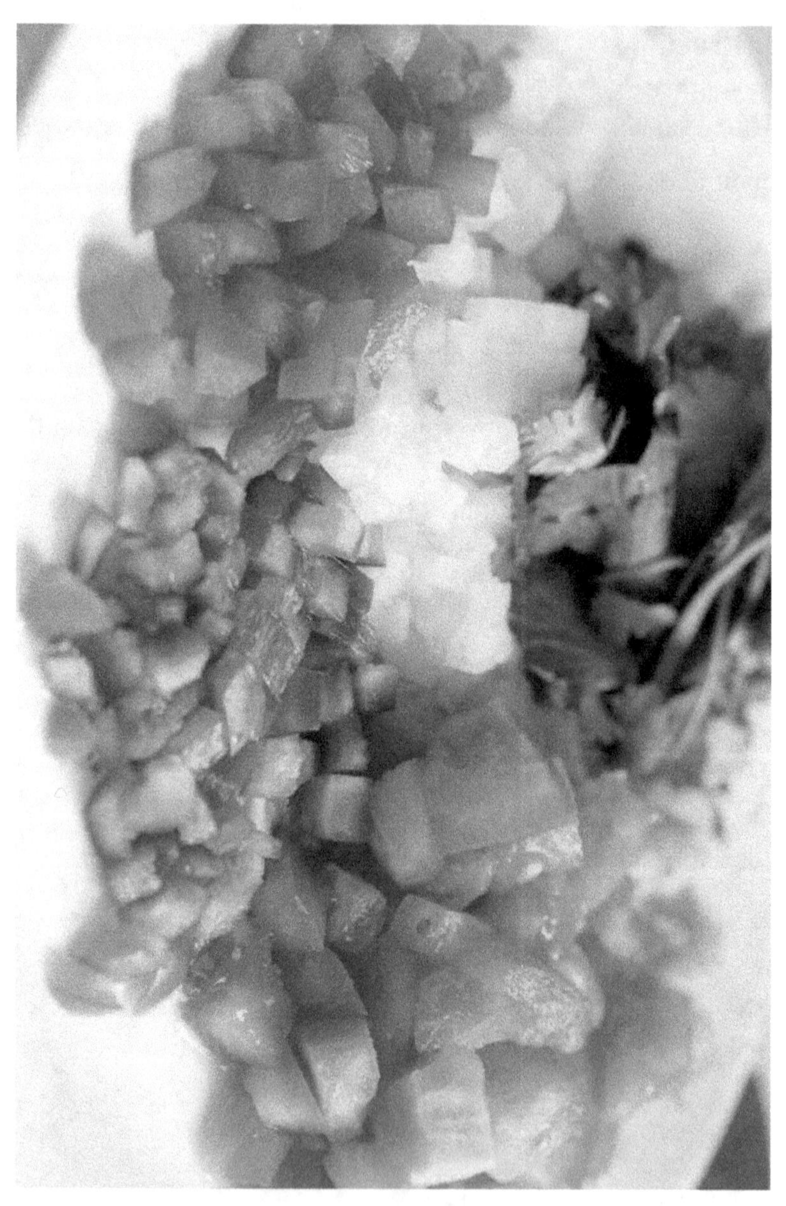

CHAPTER FOUR

Menstrual Cramp Relief Diet Dinner Recipes

1. Baked Salmon with Lemon and Dill

Salmon is rich in omega-3 fatty acids, which can help reduce inflammation and ease menstrual cramps.

Ingredients:

- 2 salmon fillets
- 1 lemon, thinly sliced
- Fresh dill
- Olive oil
- Salt and pepper to taste

Instructions:

1. Preheat your oven to 375°F (190°C).

2. Place salmon fillets on a baking sheet.

3. Drizzle with olive oil, season with salt and pepper, and top with lemon slices and fresh dill.

4. Bake for 15-20 minutes or until salmon flakes easily.

5. Serve hot!

Cooking Time: 20-25 minutes

2. Spinach and Mushroom Quiche

This quiche is packed with iron-rich spinach and mushrooms, offering relief from menstrual cramps.

Ingredients:

- 1 pie crust (store-bought or homemade)
- 2 cups fresh spinach leaves
- 1 cup sliced mushrooms
- 1/2 onion, chopped
- 4 eggs
- 1 cup milk (or milk alternative)
- 1 cup shredded cheese (e.g., Swiss, cheddar)
- Salt and pepper to taste

Instructions:

1. Preheat your oven to 375°F (190°C).

2. In a pan, sauté spinach, mushrooms, and onions until softened.

3. In a bowl, whisk together eggs, milk, shredded cheese, salt, and pepper.

4. Place the pie crust in a pie dish.

5. Spread the sautéed vegetables evenly in the crust.

6. Pour the egg mixture over the vegetables.

7. Bake for 30-35 minutes or until the quiche is set and lightly browned.

8. Allow it to cool slightly before slicing.

Cooking Time: 40-45 minutes

3. Lentil and Vegetable Stir-Fry

This stir-fry features protein-rich lentils and an array of colorful vegetables, providing essential nutrients to ease menstrual cramps.

Ingredients:

- 1 cup dried green or brown lentils
- 2 cups water
- 2 cups mixed vegetables (e.g., bell peppers, broccoli, carrots)
- 2 tablespoons soy sauce
- 1 tablespoon sesame oil
- 1 teaspoon ginger, minced
- Cooked brown rice

Instructions:

1. In a pot, combine lentils and water. Bring to a boil, then reduce heat and simmer for about 20-25 minutes or until lentils are tender. Drain any excess water.

2. Heat sesame oil in a pan or wok over medium-high heat.

3. Add mixed vegetables and ginger; stir-fry until tender-crisp.

4. Stir in cooked lentils and soy sauce.

5. Serve over cooked brown rice.

Cooking Time: 30-35 minutes (including lentil cooking time)

4. Vegetable and Chickpea Curry

This curry is loaded with vegetables and chickpeas, which provide fiber and nutrients known to relieve cramps.

Ingredients:

- 1 can (15 oz) chickpeas, drained and rinsed
- 2 cups mixed vegetables (e.g., cauliflower, bell peppers, peas)

- 1 onion, finely chopped

- 2 cloves garlic, minced

- 1 can (14 oz) diced tomatoes

- 2 tablespoons curry paste or powder

- 1 cup coconut milk

- Olive oil

- Salt and pepper to taste

Instructions:

1. In a large pan, heat olive oil over medium heat.

2. Add chopped onion and garlic; sauté until fragrant.

3. Stir in curry paste or powder and cook for another minute.

4. Add mixed vegetables and sauté for a few minutes.

5. Pour in diced tomatoes, chickpeas, and coconut milk.

6. Simmer for 15-20 minutes, or until vegetables are tender.

7. Season with salt and pepper.

8. Serve your vegetable and chickpea curry over rice or with naan bread.

Cooking Time: 30-35 minutes

5. Ginger and Turmeric Chicken Stir-Fry

Ginger and turmeric are known for their anti-inflammatory properties. This stir-fry features these spices along with chicken and vegetables for cramp relief.

Ingredients:

- 2 boneless, skinless chicken breasts, sliced
- 2 tablespoons olive oil
- 1 onion, thinly sliced
- 2 cloves garlic, minced
- 1 tablespoon fresh ginger, grated
- 1 teaspoon ground turmeric
- Mixed vegetables (e.g., bell peppers, broccoli, snap peas)
- Soy sauce
- Cooked brown rice

Instructions:

1. In a wok or large pan, heat olive oil over medium-high heat.

2. Add sliced chicken and cook until browned and cooked through. Remove from the pan and set aside.

3. In the same pan, add more oil if needed. Sauté onion, garlic, ginger, and turmeric until fragrant.

4. Add mixed vegetables and stir-fry until tender-crisp.

5. Return cooked chicken to the pan, add soy sauce to taste, and stir until everything is well combined.

6. Serve over cooked brown rice.

Cooking Time: 30-35 minutes

6. Butternut Squash and Sage Risotto

Butternut squash provides vitamins and fiber, while sage adds flavor and helps reduce cramps in this comforting risotto.

Ingredients:

- 1 cup Arborio rice
- 2 cups diced butternut squash
- 1/2 onion, finely chopped
- 2 cloves garlic, minced
- 1/2 cup dry white wine (optional)
- 4 cups vegetable broth
- Fresh sage leaves

- Parmesan cheese (optional)

- Olive oil

- Salt and pepper to taste

Instructions:

1. Heat olive oil in a large pan over medium heat.

2. Sauté chopped onion and garlic until translucent.

3. Add Arborio rice and stir until lightly toasted.

4. Pour in white wine and stir until mostly absorbed.

5. Begin adding vegetable broth one cup at a time, stirring frequently and allowing the liquid to absorb before adding more.

6. After adding two cups of broth, stir in diced butternut squash.

7. Continue adding broth and stirring until the rice and squash are tender and creamy.

8. Season with salt and pepper, and stir in fresh sage leaves.

9. Optionally, top with Parmesan cheese before serving.

Cooking Time: 40-45 minutes

7. Spaghetti Squash with Tomato and Basil Sauce

This dish substitutes traditional pasta with spaghetti squash, providing a lower-carb option while still enjoying a flavorful tomato and basil sauce.

Ingredients:

- 1 spaghetti squash
- 2 cups tomato sauce (store-bought or homemade)
- Fresh basil leaves
- Olive oil
- Salt and pepper to taste
- Grated Parmesan cheese (optional)

Instructions:

1. Preheat your oven to 375°F (190°C).

2. Cut the spaghetti squash in half lengthwise and scoop out the seeds.

3. Drizzle olive oil over the cut sides and season with salt and pepper.

4. Place the squash halves cut-side down on a baking sheet and bake for 35-40 minutes, or until the flesh easily shreds into "spaghetti" with a fork.

5. While the squash is baking, heat tomato sauce in a pan over low heat.

6. Once the squash is done, use a fork to scrape the flesh into "spaghetti" strands.

7. Serve the squash with tomato sauce, fresh basil leaves, and grated Parmesan cheese if desired.

Cooking Time: 45-50 minutes

8. Tofu and Vegetable Curry

This flavorful curry features tofu for protein and a medley of vegetables, offering cramp relief in a delicious and spicy package.

Ingredients:

- 1 block firm tofu, cubed
- 2 cups mixed vegetables (e.g., bell peppers, cauliflower, snap peas)
- 1 onion, chopped

- 2 cloves garlic, minced

- 1 can (14 oz) coconut milk

- 2 tablespoons red curry paste

- Olive oil

- Salt and pepper to taste

Instructions:

1. In a large pan, heat olive oil over medium heat.

2. Add chopped onion and garlic; sauté until fragrant.

3. Stir in red curry paste and cook for another minute.

4. Add mixed vegetables and sauté for a few minutes.

5. Add cubed tofu and coconut milk.

6. Simmer for 15-20 minutes, or until vegetables are tender.

7. Season with salt and pepper.

8. Serve your tofu and vegetable curry over rice or with naan bread.

Cooking Time: 30-35 minutes

9. Mediterranean Stuffed Bell Peppers

These stuffed bell peppers are filled with quinoa, chickpeas, and a variety of Mediterranean-inspired ingredients for a wholesome dinner.

Ingredients:

- 4 bell peppers, halved and seeds removed
- 1 cup cooked quinoa
- 1 can (15 oz) chickpeas, drained and rinsed
- Cherry tomatoes, halved
- Cucumber, diced
- Kalamata olives, pitted and sliced
- Feta cheese (optional)
- Olive oil
- Salt and pepper to taste

Instructions:

1. Preheat your oven to 375°F (190°C).

2. Place bell pepper halves in a baking dish and drizzle with olive oil. Season with salt and pepper.

3. In a bowl, combine cooked quinoa, chickpeas, cherry

tomatoes, cucumber, and Kalamata olives.

4. Stuff each bell pepper half with the quinoa and chickpea mixture.

5. Optionally, top with crumbled feta cheese.

6. Cover the baking dish with foil and bake for 25-30 minutes, or until the peppers are tender.

7. Serve hot!

Cooking Time: 30-35 minutes

10. Eggplant Parmesan

This vegetarian dish features eggplant for fiber and nutrients, layered with marinara sauce and cheese for a comforting and cramp-relieving dinner.

Ingredients:

- 2 large eggplants, sliced into rounds
- 2 cups marinara sauce (store-bought or homemade)
- 1 cup shredded mozzarella cheese
- 1/2 cup grated Parmesan cheese
- Fresh basil leaves

- Olive oil

- Salt and pepper to taste

Instructions:

1. Preheat your oven to 375°F (190°C).

2. Place eggplant slices on a baking sheet, drizzle with olive oil, and season with salt and pepper.

3. Bake eggplant slices for about 15 minutes, or until tender.

4. In a baking dish, layer marinara sauce, eggplant slices, mozzarella cheese, and grated Parmesan cheese.

5. Repeat the layers as needed, finishing with a cheese layer on top.

6. Bake uncovered for 25-30 minutes, or until the cheese is bubbly and golden.

7. Garnish with fresh basil leaves before serving.

Cooking Time: 40-45 minutes

Menstrual Cramp Relief Diet Snacks Recipes

1. Greek Yogurt and Berry Parfait

This parfait is packed with calcium from Greek yogurt and antioxidants from berries, which can help alleviate cramps.

Ingredients:

- 1 cup Greek yogurt
- 1/2 cup mixed berries (e.g., strawberries, blueberries, raspberries)
- 1 tablespoon honey (optional)
- A handful of granola

Instructions:

1. In a glass or bowl, layer Greek yogurt, mixed berries, and granola.

2. Drizzle with honey if desired.

3. Repeat for additional servings.

4. Enjoy your parfait!

Preparation Time: 5 minutes

2. Hummus and Veggie Sticks

This snack pairs creamy hummus with fresh vegetable sticks for a nutritious and cramp-relieving option.

Ingredients:

- 1/2 cup hummus (store-bought or homemade)
- Baby carrots, cucumber sticks, and bell pepper strips

Instructions:

1. Place hummus in a small bowl.

2. Arrange vegetable sticks on a plate.

3. Dip and enjoy!

Preparation Time: 5 minutes

3. Peanut Butter and Banana Bites

These bite-sized snacks combine potassium-rich bananas with peanut butter for a delicious and cramp-relieving treat.

Ingredients:

- 1 banana, sliced
- 2 tablespoons peanut butter

- Optional toppings: chia seeds, honey, or chopped nuts

Instructions:

1. Spread peanut butter on banana slices.

2. Optionally, sprinkle with chia seeds, drizzle with honey, or add chopped nuts.

3. Serve and enjoy!

Preparation Time: 5 minutes

4. Cottage Cheese and Pineapple Cups

Cottage cheese provides protein and calcium, while pineapple offers bromelain, known for its anti-inflammatory properties.

Ingredients:

- 1 cup cottage cheese
- 1 cup fresh pineapple chunks

Instructions:

1. In a bowl or cup, layer cottage cheese and pineapple

chunks.

2. Repeat for additional servings.

3. Enjoy your cottage cheese and pineapple cups!

Preparation Time: 5 minutes

5. Almond Butter and Apple Slices

Almond butter is rich in healthy fats and protein, making it a satisfying snack when paired with apple slices.

Ingredients:

- 2 tablespoons almond butter
- 1 apple, sliced

Instructions:

1. Spread almond butter on apple slices.

2. Enjoy your almond butter and apple snack!

Preparation Time: 5 minutes

6. Trail Mix with Dark Chocolate

This trail mix combines nuts, seeds, and dark chocolate, providing magnesium and antioxidants to help relieve cramps.

Ingredients:

- 1/2 cup mixed nuts (e.g., almonds, walnuts, cashews)
- 2 tablespoons pumpkin seeds
- 2 tablespoons sunflower seeds
- 2 tablespoons dark chocolate chips

Instructions:

1. Mix all the ingredients in a bowl.

2. Portion into small snack-sized bags for easy access.

3. Enjoy your trail mix!

Preparation Time:5 minutes

7. Chia Seed Pudding

Chia seeds are packed with fiber and omega-3s, which can help reduce inflammation and cramps.

Ingredients:

- 2 tablespoons chia seeds
- 1/2 cup almond milk

- 1/2 teaspoon vanilla extract

- 1/2 teaspoon honey (optional)

- Fresh berries for topping

Instructions:

1. In a jar or bowl, mix chia seeds, almond milk, vanilla extract, and honey (if desired).

2. Stir well, cover, and refrigerate for at least 2 hours or overnight to thicken.

3. Top with fresh berries before serving.

4. Enjoy your chia pudding!

Preparation Time: 2 hours (mostly refrigeration time)

8. Popcorn with Nutritional Yeast

Popcorn is a whole grain, and nutritional yeast adds a cheesy flavor and extra nutrients to this easy snack.

Ingredients:

- 2 cups popped popcorn

- 2 tablespoons nutritional yeast

- Salt and pepper to taste

Instructions:

1. Pop the popcorn according to package instructions.

2. Sprinkle nutritional yeast, salt, and pepper over the popped popcorn.

3. Toss to coat evenly.

4. Enjoy your cheesy popcorn!

Preparation Time: 10 minutes (including popcorn popping)

9. Frozen Grapes

Frozen grapes are a simple and refreshing snack, offering natural sweetness and hydration.

Ingredients:

- Fresh grapes (red or green)

Instructions:

1. Wash and dry grapes.

2. Place them in the freezer for at least 2 hours.

3. Enjoy your frozen grapes!

Preparation Time: 2 hours (freezing time)

10. Cucumber and Tzatziki Dip

Cucumber slices paired with creamy tzatziki dip make for a cooling and cramp-relieving snack.

Ingredients:

- 1 cucumber, sliced
- 1/2 cup tzatziki sauce (store-bought or homemade)

Instructions:

1. Arrange cucumber slices on a plate.

2. Serve with tzatziki sauce for dipping.

3. Enjoy your cucumber and tzatziki snack!

Preparation Time: 5 minutes

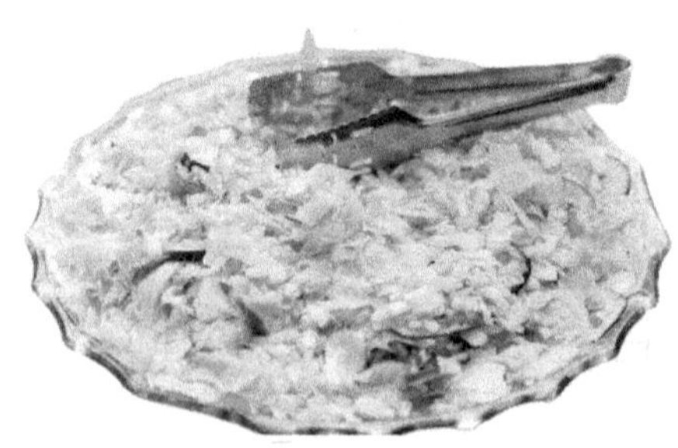

CONCLUSION

In conclusion, adopting a menstrual cramp relief diet can be a proactive and effective approach for individuals seeking natural ways to alleviate the discomfort associated with menstruation. This dietary strategy revolves around incorporating specific foods and nutrients that have been scientifically linked to reducing inflammation, easing muscle tension, and balancing hormonal fluctuations.

By prioritizing foods rich in magnesium, calcium, omega-3 fatty acids, and anti-inflammatory compounds, individuals can potentially experience a reduction in the severity and duration of menstrual cramps. These foods include leafy greens, fatty fish, nuts, seeds, whole grains, and various fruits and vegetables.

Additionally, staying well-hydrated and avoiding excessive salt and caffeine intake can help manage bloating and water retention during the menstrual cycle.

Furthermore, embracing a menstrual cramp relief diet doesn't have to mean sacrificing taste or variety in your meals. The provided meal plans and recipes demonstrate that it is possible to enjoy delicious and nutritious dishes while also supporting menstrual health. From nutrient-packed breakfasts to satisfying dinners and even indulgent snacks, there are plenty of options to cater to individual tastes and preferences. It's essential to remember that dietary changes may not yield immediate results and may vary in effectiveness from person to person.

Patience and consistency are key when adopting a new dietary approach. Consulting with a healthcare professional or nutritionist is also advisable, especially for individuals with specific dietary requirements or underlying health conditions.

Ultimately, a menstrual cramp relief diet is just one piece of the puzzle when it comes to managing menstrual discomfort. Incorporating regular physical activity, practicing stress-reduction techniques, and ensuring adequate sleep are also vital components of a holistic approach to menstrual health.

By combining these strategies, individuals can empower themselves to better navigate their menstrual cycles and experience fewer disruptions in their daily lives, ultimately enhancing their overall well-being and quality of life.